ARTESUNATE

Guide :Artwell-60

Comprehensive Protocols for Malaria Treatment

Dr. Mason Hudson

Table of Contents

Chapter 1: 7

    INTRODUCTION AND BASIC INFORMATION 7

        Description 8

        Pharmacology 10

        Microbiology 11

Chapter 2: 14

    CLINICAL INFORMATION 14

        Pharmacokinetics 14

        Contraindications 19

        Precautions 21

        Usage in Pregnancy 23

Chapter 3: 26

INTERACTIONS AND ADVERSE EFFECTS............26

Drug Interactions...26

1. Antimalarials:..26

2. Antiretrovirals:..28

3. Anticonvulsants: 29

4. Anticoagulants:..30

Adverse Effects 31

1. Common Adverse Effects: 31

2. Hematologic Effects:....................................32

3. Cardiotoxicity:..33

Management of Adverse Effects: 37

Chapter 4: 39

ADMINISTRATION AND DOSAGE 39

Dosage and Administration 39

Duration of Therapy 42

Method of Administration 44

Combination Therapy 47

Common Combinations: 48

Overdose 50

2. Management of Overdose: 51

3. Preventive Measures: 53

Chapter 5: 54

ADDITIONAL INFORMATION 54

Preclinical Data 54

1. Pharmacodynamics: 54

3. Toxicology: 57

Storage 59

Instructions 62

Presentation 66

Chapter 1:
INTRODUCTION AND BASIC INFORMATION

Composition

Artesunate is a water-soluble hemisuccinate derivative of dihydroartemisinin, which itself is derived from artemisinin, a compound extracted from the sweet wormwood plant (Artemisia annua). The artesunate injection typically consists of the active ingredient, artesunate, along with other excipients that stabilize the formulation. The exact composition may vary slightly depending on the manufacturer, but a standard preparation might include the following components:

Active Ingredient: Artesunate ($C_{19}H_{28}O_8$) is the primary active component. It is a white or almost white powder that is freely soluble in water.

Solvent: Usually, a solvent such as sodium bicarbonate or phosphate buffer is included to reconstitute the artesunate powder into an injectable form.

Stabilizers and Preservatives: These might include substances such as ethanol, glycerin, or benzyl alcohol to ensure the stability and sterility of the solution.

The typical formulation involves reconstituting the artesunate powder with the provided solvent to produce a solution ready for intravenous or intramuscular injection. The concentration of artesunate in the final solution is usually adjusted to provide the necessary therapeutic dose.

Description

Artesunate is an antimalarial agent used primarily for the treatment of severe malaria caused by Plasmodium falciparum, a parasite known for its resistance to many other antimalarial drugs. Its chemical structure is characterized by an endoperoxide bridge, which is crucial for its antimalarial activity. Artesunate is a derivative of artemisinin, a traditional Chinese medicine known for its potent and rapid antimalarial effects.

The drug is presented as a lyophilized powder for injection, which requires reconstitution with a specific solvent before administration. Upon reconstitution, it forms a clear, colorless solution suitable for intravenous or intramuscular injection. Artesunate is known for its rapid action, significantly reducing the parasite load within hours of administration, which is critical in severe malaria cases where quick intervention can be life-saving.

Pharmacology

The pharmacological activity of artesunate is largely attributed to its ability to generate reactive oxygen species (ROS) and free radicals. These reactive molecules cause extensive damage to the proteins and cellular membranes of the malaria parasite, leading to its death. The key pharmacological properties include:

Mechanism of Action: Artesunate acts by interacting with the iron in the parasite's heme group, leading to the generation of ROS. These reactive species attack the parasite's cellular components, causing oxidative stress and damage that ultimately kill the parasite.

Rapid Action: One of the most significant advantages of artesunate is its rapid onset of action. After administration, artesunate quickly reduces the parasite biomass, which is crucial in severe malaria cases where high parasite loads can cause life-threatening complications.

Conversion to Active Metabolite: In the body, artesunate is rapidly converted to its active metabolite, dihydroartemisinin (DHA). DHA is responsible for the drug's potent antimalarial effects and has a half-life of approximately 1-2 hours, facilitating its quick action and effective parasite clearance.

Efficacy Against Drug-Resistant Strains: Artesunate is effective against multi-drug resistant strains of Plasmodium falciparum, making it an essential tool in regions where resistance to other antimalarials is prevalent.

Microbiology

Artesunate primarily targets the asexual erythrocytic stages of Plasmodium parasites, the stage responsible for the clinical symptoms of malaria. Its effectiveness against Plasmodium falciparum, the most dangerous malaria parasite species, is well-documented, but it also has activity against other species such as Plasmodium vivax, Plasmodium ovale, and Plasmodium malariae.

Mode of Action in Microorganisms: Artesunate disrupts the parasite's mitochondrial function and inhibits protein synthesis. The generation of ROS and the ensuing oxidative damage are critical to its mode of action. Additionally, artesunate interferes with the parasite's ability to detoxify free heme, a toxic byproduct of hemoglobin digestion, leading to its accumulation and parasite death.

Spectrum of Activity: While primarily used for malaria, artesunate also shows activity against other parasitic infections and has been explored for its potential use in treating certain types of cancer and viral infections, owing to its ability to induce apoptosis and inhibit cell proliferation.

Resistance Patterns: Although resistance to artemisinin derivatives has been reported, particularly in the Greater Mekong Subregion, artesunate remains effective in many parts of the world. Resistance mechanisms typically involve mutations in the K13 gene, which affect the parasite's response to the drug. Ongoing research aims to understand and combat these resistance mechanisms to ensure the continued efficacy of artesunate.

Chapter 2:

CLINICAL INFORMATION

Pharmacokinetics

Absorption

Artesunate is typically administered intravenously (IV) or intramuscularly (IM), allowing for rapid absorption and onset of action. When given IV, artesunate is almost immediately available in the bloodstream, which is crucial for treating severe malaria cases. IM administration also ensures rapid absorption, although it may be slightly slower compared to IV administration.

Distribution

Following administration, artesunate is rapidly converted to its active metabolite, dihydroartemisinin (DHA). DHA is distributed widely throughout the body, with particularly high concentrations found in the liver, spleen, kidneys, and lungs. The volume of distribution is relatively high, indicating extensive tissue penetration, which is essential for effectively targeting malaria parasites throughout the body. The plasma protein binding of DHA is around 93%, suggesting that a significant proportion of the drug remains free and active in the bloodstream.

Metabolism

Artesunate undergoes rapid hydrolysis by plasma esterases to form DHA, the primary active metabolite responsible for its antimalarial effects. DHA is further metabolized through glucuronidation by the liver. The rapid conversion of artesunate to DHA ensures quick therapeutic effects, which is critical in severe malaria where timely parasite clearance can be life-saving.

Excretion

The metabolites of DHA are primarily excreted through the urine. The elimination half-life of DHA is approximately 1-2 hours, meaning the drug is cleared relatively quickly from the body. However, the rapid action and short half-life necessitate repeated dosing to maintain effective therapeutic levels, particularly in severe malaria cases.

Special Populations

Pharmacokinetic studies have shown that artesunate and DHA are processed similarly in adults and children, making the drug suitable for pediatric use. However, patients with severe renal or hepatic impairment may exhibit altered pharmacokinetics, necessitating close monitoring and possible dose adjustments.

Indications

Artesunate is indicated primarily for the treatment of severe malaria, particularly when caused by Plasmodium falciparum. Due to its rapid action and effectiveness against drug-resistant strains, it is the preferred treatment in many endemic regions. Specific indications include:

Severe Malaria: Artesunate is the first-line treatment for severe malaria, which can present with complications such as cerebral malaria, severe anemia, respiratory distress, and organ failure. It is effective in rapidly reducing the parasite biomass and preventing further complications.

Uncomplicated Malaria: Although primarily used for severe cases, artesunate can also be used for uncomplicated malaria, particularly when caused by Plasmodium falciparum and in areas with high levels of drug resistance. It is often used in combination with other antimalarial drugs to ensure complete parasite clearance and reduce the risk of resistance development.

Multidrug-Resistant Malaria: Artesunate is highly effective against malaria strains resistant to other antimalarial drugs such as chloroquine, sulfadoxine-pyrimethamine, and mefloquine. Its use in areas with high levels of drug resistance helps to maintain treatment efficacy and control malaria transmission.

Malaria in Pregnancy: Artesunate is considered safe and effective for the treatment of severe malaria in pregnant women, particularly in the second and third trimesters. Its rapid action and effectiveness are crucial in preventing severe complications for both the mother and the fetus.

Contraindications

While artesunate is generally safe and well-tolerated, there are certain conditions where its use is contraindicated or requires caution:

Hypersensitivity: Patients with known hypersensitivity to artesunate or any of its components should not receive the drug. Hypersensitivity reactions can include rash, urticaria, and anaphylaxis, which require immediate discontinuation of the drug and appropriate medical intervention.

Severe Renal or Hepatic Impairment: Patients with severe renal or hepatic impairment may require dose adjustments and close monitoring due to altered pharmacokinetics and the potential for accumulation of the drug or its metabolites.

First Trimester of Pregnancy: Although artesunate is generally considered safe in pregnancy, its use in the first trimester should be carefully weighed against the risks. Animal studies have shown some potential for embryotoxicity, and while human data are limited, the risks and benefits must be considered on a case-by-case basis.

Co-Administration with Certain Drugs: Artesunate should be used cautiously with drugs that may interact adversely, such as other antimalarials, anticoagulants, and certain anticonvulsants. Drug interactions can alter the effectiveness and safety profile of artesunate, necessitating careful consideration of co-administered medications.

Precautions

Several precautions should be considered when administering artesunate to ensure patient safety and optimize therapeutic outcomes:

Monitoring for Adverse Reactions: Patients receiving artesunate should be closely monitored for adverse reactions, particularly hypersensitivity reactions. Regular monitoring of vital signs, liver and kidney function, and complete blood counts is recommended to detect any potential complications early.

Avoiding Resistance: To minimize the risk of developing drug resistance, artesunate should be used in combination with other antimalarial drugs as part of a combination therapy regimen. Monotherapy can lead to the selection of resistant parasites, reducing the long-term efficacy of the drug.

Patient Education: Patients and caregivers should be educated on the importance of completing the full course of treatment, even if symptoms improve before the medication is finished. This helps ensure complete parasite clearance and reduces the risk of resistance.

Use in Pediatric Patients: Artesunate is safe and effective for use in children, including infants. However, dosing should be carefully calculated based on body weight to ensure therapeutic efficacy and minimize the risk of adverse effects.

Pregnancy Considerations: For pregnant women, particularly those in the first trimester, the risks and benefits of artesunate use should be carefully considered. While the drug is crucial for treating severe malaria, potential risks to the fetus must be weighed against the dangers of untreated malaria.

Usage in Pregnancy

Malaria in pregnancy poses significant risks to both the mother and the fetus, including severe anemia, low birth weight, premature delivery, and increased mortality. Therefore, effective treatment is critical. Artesunate is one of the preferred treatments for severe malaria in pregnant women due to its rapid action and effectiveness against drug-resistant strains.

First Trimester: The use of artesunate in the first trimester should be approached with caution. Although animal studies have indicated potential risks, the benefits of treating severe malaria, which can be life-threatening, often outweigh the potential risks. The decision to use artesunate during this period should involve careful consideration of the clinical situation and consultation with a specialist.

Second and Third Trimesters: Artesunate is considered safe and effective during the second and third trimesters. The risk of severe malaria complications during these stages of pregnancy is high, and prompt treatment with artesunate can prevent maternal and fetal morbidity and mortality. The drug's rapid action helps to quickly reduce the parasite load, which is crucial for the health of both the mother and the developing fetus.

Postpartum Considerations: Following delivery, women who were treated with artesunate during pregnancy should continue to be monitored for any delayed adverse effects. Additionally, breastfeeding mothers can safely continue to use artesunate if needed, as the drug and its metabolites are excreted in breast milk in very small amounts that are not harmful to the infant.

Prevention of Malaria in Pregnancy: While artesunate is used for the treatment of malaria, preventing malaria in pregnancy is equally important. Pregnant women in endemic areas should use preventive measures such as insecticide-treated bed nets, indoor residual spraying, and intermittent preventive treatment with sulfadoxine-pyrimethamine (IPTp-SP) as recommended by WHO guidelines.

Chapter 3:

INTERACTIONS AND ADVERSE EFFECTS

Drug Interactions

Artesunate, like many medications, can interact with other drugs, potentially affecting its efficacy or increasing the risk of adverse effects. Understanding these interactions is crucial for ensuring safe and effective treatment, particularly in regions where polypharmacy is common due to co-infections or multiple health conditions.

1. Antimalarials:

Artesunate is often used in combination with other antimalarial drugs to enhance efficacy and prevent resistance. However, interactions with these drugs can influence treatment outcomes:

Artemether-Lumefantrine: Combination therapies like artemether-lumefantrine can enhance the antimalarial efficacy. However, both drugs prolong the QT interval, raising concerns about additive effects leading to arrhythmias. Monitoring cardiac function is recommended during co-administration.

Quinine: Co-administration with quinine may lead to increased risk of cardiac toxicity. Artesunate-quinine combination is generally avoided unless absolutely necessary, and even then, with careful monitoring.

Doxycycline and Clindamycin: These antibiotics are sometimes used alongside artesunate to treat malaria. They have no significant pharmacokinetic interactions, making them safe options to enhance antimalarial treatment.

2. Antiretrovirals:

In malaria-endemic regions with high HIV prevalence, patients often require both antimalarials and antiretrovirals (ARVs). Significant interactions include:

Protease Inhibitors (PIs): Drugs like ritonavir can inhibit CYP3A4, the enzyme responsible for metabolizing DHA. This can lead to increased levels of DHA, potentially enhancing both efficacy and toxicity. Dose adjustments and close monitoring may be necessary.

Non-Nucleoside Reverse Transcriptase Inhibitors (NNRTIs): Drugs like efavirenz can induce CYP3A4, potentially reducing DHA levels and efficacy. Adjustments to artesunate dosage or alternative malaria treatment options might be required.

3. Anticonvulsants:

Certain anticonvulsants, particularly those that induce or inhibit CYP enzymes, can interact with artesunate:

Carbamazepine and Phenytoin: These drugs are potent CYP3A4 inducers, potentially reducing artesunate and DHA levels, leading to subtherapeutic concentrations and treatment failure. Alternative anticonvulsants or adjusted dosing may be necessary.

4. Anticoagulants:

Warfarin, a commonly used anticoagulant, has a narrow therapeutic index and is metabolized by CYP2C9, which can be inhibited by DHA:

Warfarin: Co-administration may increase warfarin levels, enhancing anticoagulant effects and bleeding risk. Frequent monitoring of INR (International Normalized Ratio) and warfarin dose adjustments are essential.

5. Other Considerations:

Herbal Supplements: Patients may use traditional herbal medicines, some of which can interact with artesunate. For example, St.

John's Wort, a CYP3A4 inducer, may reduce DHA levels.

CYP3A4 Inhibitors/Inducers: Other drugs that inhibit or induce CYP3A4 can affect artesunate metabolism. Grapefruit juice, for example, is a known CYP3A4 inhibitor that can increase DHA levels.

Adverse Effects

Artesunate is generally well-tolerated, but like all medications, it can cause side effects. Understanding these adverse effects is critical for managing and mitigating risks during treatment.

1. Common Adverse Effects:

Gastrointestinal Disturbances: Nausea, vomiting, diarrhea, and abdominal pain are relatively common. These effects are usually mild to moderate and resolve without specific treatment.

Headache and Dizziness: These are also common and typically transient. They can be managed with symptomatic treatment and do not usually necessitate discontinuation of therapy.

2. Hematologic Effects:

Anemia: Artesunate can cause hemolytic anemia, particularly in patients with G6PD deficiency. Monitoring hemoglobin levels during treatment is essential. In severe cases, blood transfusions may be necessary.

Neutropenia: A decrease in neutrophil counts can occur, increasing the risk of infections.

Regular blood counts are recommended during treatment, and any signs of infection should be promptly addressed.

3. Cardiotoxicity:

QT Prolongation: Artesunate, particularly in combination with other QT-prolonging drugs, can cause QT interval prolongation, increasing the risk of arrhythmias. ECG monitoring is recommended in patients with cardiac conditions or those on concurrent QT-prolonging medications.

4. Neurotoxicity:

Dizziness and Seizures: Neurotoxic effects, including dizziness and seizures, have been reported, particularly at higher doses or prolonged treatment. Patients with a history of seizures should be closely monitored.

5. Allergic Reactions:

Hypersensitivity: Rash, urticaria, and anaphylaxis are potential allergic reactions to artesunate. Immediate discontinuation and appropriate medical intervention are required in such cases.

6. Injection Site Reactions:

Pain and Inflammation: IM administration can cause local pain, swelling, and inflammation at the injection site. Proper injection technique and rotation of injection sites can help minimize these effects.

7. Liver and Kidney Effects:

Hepatotoxicity: Elevated liver enzymes and, rarely, jaundice can occur. Liver function should be monitored, particularly in patients with pre-existing liver conditions.

Nephrotoxicity: Although rare, artesunate can affect kidney function, particularly in patients with underlying renal impairment. Monitoring renal function during treatment is advised.

8. Hemolysis and Delayed Hemolysis:

Acute Hemolysis: Acute hemolysis, particularly in patients with G6PD deficiency, can occur soon after treatment initiation.

Delayed Hemolysis: Delayed hemolysis has been reported, usually occurring weeks after treatment completion. Patients should be informed about this risk and monitored for signs of hemolysis, such as fatigue, pallor, and jaundice.

9. Impact on the Immune System:

Immunosuppression: Artesunate can have immunosuppressive effects, potentially increasing susceptibility to infections. Monitoring for signs of infection and appropriate prophylactic measures are recommended.

10. Effects on Pregnancy and Fetus:

Teratogenicity: Although artesunate is considered safe in the second and third trimesters, animal studies have shown potential teratogenic effects. Human data are limited, but caution is advised, particularly in the first trimester.

Fetal Hemolysis: Artesunate can cross the placenta, potentially causing hemolysis in the fetus, especially in cases of maternal G6PD deficiency.

11. Long-Term Effects:

No significant long-term adverse effects have been associated with artesunate, but long-term safety data are limited. Continued monitoring and reporting of any long-term adverse effects are essential for comprehensive safety profiling.

Management of Adverse Effects:

Symptomatic Treatment: Mild to moderate adverse effects, such as gastrointestinal disturbances and headaches, can often be managed with symptomatic treatment and do not require discontinuation of artesunate.

Dose Adjustment: In cases of severe adverse effects, dose adjustments or switching to an alternative antimalarial may be necessary. This decision should be based on a careful assessment of the risk-benefit ratio.

Monitoring: Regular monitoring of blood counts, liver and kidney function, and cardiac function (ECG) can help detect and manage adverse effects early, minimizing the risk of serious complications.

Patient Education: Educating patients about potential adverse effects and the importance of reporting any unusual symptoms promptly can help manage and mitigate risks effectivel

Chapter 4:

ADMINISTRATION AND DOSAGE

Dosage and Administration

The correct dosage and administration of artesunate are critical for its effectiveness in treating malaria, especially severe cases. Proper administration ensures rapid parasite clearance and minimizes the risk of resistance and adverse effects.

1. Intravenous (IV) Administration:

Dosage: The standard dosage for IV administration of artesunate in adults and children weighing over 20 kg is 2.4 mg/kg body weight per dose. The regimen typically involves an initial dose at 0 hours, followed by additional doses at 12 and 24 hours, and then once daily until the patient can tolerate oral medication or for a maximum of 7 days.

Preparation: Artesunate is supplied as a lyophilized powder that must be reconstituted with the accompanying diluent or a suitable solvent (such as 5% dextrose or normal saline) to achieve the desired concentration. Typically, 1 vial of artesunate (60 mg) is reconstituted with 1 ml of diluent to produce a 60 mg/ml solution.

Administration: After reconstitution, the artesunate solution should be administered slowly via IV injection over 1-2 minutes. Alternatively, it can be diluted further and administered as an IV infusion over 30 minutes to an hour.

2. Intramuscular (IM) Administration:

Dosage: The IM dosage is identical to the IV regimen, at 2.4 mg/kg body weight per dose, following the same schedule of 0, 12, and 24 hours, and then daily.

Preparation: Similar to IV administration, artesunate must be reconstituted. For IM administration, the reconstituted solution is drawn into a syringe and injected deep into a large muscle, typically the thigh or buttock.

Administration: The injection should be administered slowly to minimize pain and tissue damage. Rotating injection sites can help reduce local adverse reactions.

3. Pediatric Dosage:

Infants and Children under 20 kg: The dosage is typically 3 mg/kg body weight per dose to account for differences in drug metabolism and distribution in younger patients. The same administration schedule is followed.

Neonates and Premature Infants: Artesunate is safe for use in neonates and premature infants, but the dosage must be carefully calculated and closely monitored due to the immature metabolic pathways in these patients.

Duration of Therapy

The duration of artesunate therapy depends on the severity of the malaria infection and the patient's response to treatment.

1. Severe Malaria:

Initial Phase: For severe malaria, artesunate is administered for at least 24 hours (three doses at 0, 12, and 24 hours).

Follow-Up Phase: After the initial 24-hour period, treatment continues daily until the patient can switch to an oral antimalarial, such as artemisinin-based combination therapy (ACT). This transition typically occurs within 2-3 days but may extend up to 7 days depending on clinical improvement and parasite clearance.

2. Uncomplicated Malaria:

Shorter Course: For uncomplicated malaria, artesunate is often used as part of an ACT regimen for 3 days. The duration and dosage may vary based on the specific combination therapy used.

3. Drug-Resistant Malaria:

Extended Therapy: In areas with high levels of drug resistance, extended therapy may be necessary to ensure complete parasite clearance. This can involve 5-7 days of artesunate treatment followed by ACT.

Method of Administration

The method of administration is crucial for ensuring the optimal therapeutic effect of artesunate. Both IV and IM routes are effective, but the choice depends on the clinical situation and available resources.

1. Intravenous Administration:

Preferred for Severe Cases: IV administration is preferred for patients with severe malaria, especially those with impaired consciousness, vomiting, or severe gastrointestinal symptoms that prevent oral administration.

Reconstitution and Dilution: After reconstitution, the solution must be used within 1 hour to ensure stability and efficacy. If not used immediately, it should be stored in a refrigerator and used within 24 hours.

Infusion: For patients who require fluid resuscitation, artesunate can be diluted in a larger volume of IV fluid and infused slowly.

2. Intramuscular Administration:

Alternative When IV Access Is Unavailable: IM administration is useful when IV access is not possible, such as in remote settings or in young children where IV cannulation is challenging.

Injection Technique: Proper technique is important to minimize pain and tissue damage. The needle should be long enough to reach deep muscle tissue, and the injection should be administered slowly.

3. Oral Transition:

Switching to Oral Therapy: Once the patient is stable and able to tolerate oral medications, the switch to oral ACT is recommended. This transition ensures continued parasite clearance and reduces the risk of recurrence.

Combination Therapy

Combination therapy is essential to enhance the efficacy of artesunate and prevent the development of resistance. Artesunate is often used in combination with other antimalarial drugs as part of ACT.

1. Artemisinin-Based Combination Therapy (ACT):

Rationale: ACT combines artesunate with a partner drug that has a longer half-life. This combination provides a synergistic effect, enhances parasite clearance, and reduces the risk of resistance.

Common Combinations:

Artesunate-Amodiaquine: Effective against uncomplicated malaria, providing rapid parasite clearance and reducing transmission.

Artesunate-Mefloquine: Used in areas with high resistance to other drugs, offering a high cure rate and extended protection.

Artesunate-Lumefantrine: A widely used combination that is highly effective and well-tolerated, suitable for both adults and children.

2. Sequential Therapy:

Severe Cases: In severe malaria, artesunate is administered first to rapidly reduce parasite load, followed by a full course of ACT to ensure complete clearance and prevent recrudescence.

Advantages: This sequential approach leverages the rapid action of artesunate and the prolonged effect of the partner drug, ensuring comprehensive treatment.

3. Resistance Management:

Preventing Resistance: Combination therapy helps prevent the development of resistance by attacking the parasite through different mechanisms. Artesunate disrupts the parasite's redox homeostasis, while the partner drug targets other aspects of parasite metabolism.

Monitoring and Adaptation: Regular monitoring of treatment efficacy and resistance patterns is crucial. Adjusting combination regimens based on local resistance data helps maintain treatment effectiveness.

Overdose

Overdose of artesunate, although rare, can occur and requires prompt management to mitigate adverse effects.

1. Symptoms of Overdose:

Gastrointestinal Symptoms: Nausea, vomiting, abdominal pain, and diarrhea are common in overdose situations.

Neurological Symptoms: Dizziness, headache, seizures, and altered mental status can occur, particularly with high doses.

Cardiotoxicity: QT prolongation and cardiac arrhythmias are serious concerns in overdose cases. Continuous ECG monitoring is recommended.

Hematologic Effects: Severe hemolysis, particularly in G6PD-deficient patients, can lead to anemia and jaundice.

2. Management of Overdose:

Immediate Supportive Care: Initial management focuses on supportive care, including airway protection, hemodynamic support, and monitoring of vital signs.

Gastrointestinal Decontamination: Activated charcoal may be administered if the overdose is recent and the patient is conscious, to reduce drug absorption.

Monitoring and Interventions: Continuous monitoring of cardiac function, blood counts, and electrolytes is essential. Intravenous fluids, electrolytes, and blood transfusions may be necessary.

Anticonvulsants: If seizures occur, anticonvulsants such as diazepam or lorazepam may be administered to control symptoms.

Hemodialysis: In severe cases, hemodialysis may be considered to remove artesunate from the bloodstream, although its effectiveness is variable due to the rapid metabolism and distribution of the drug.

3. Preventive Measures:

Accurate Dosing: Ensuring accurate dosing based on body weight is critical to prevent overdose. Careful calculation and double-checking of doses can help avoid errors.

Education and Awareness: Educating healthcare providers and caregivers about the correct dosing and administration of artesunate can reduce the risk of overdose.

Clear instructions and protocols should be followed.

Storage and Handling: Proper storage and handling of artesunate to prevent accidental overdose, particularly in pediatric settings where children may access medication, is essential.

Chapter 5:

ADDITIONAL INFORMATION

Preclinical Data

Preclinical studies of artesunate provide critical insights into its pharmacodynamics, pharmacokinetics, safety profile, and potential mechanisms of action. These studies form the foundation for clinical trials and eventual therapeutic use in humans.

1. Pharmacodynamics:

Mechanism of Action: Artesunate, a derivative of artemisinin, exerts its antimalarial effects primarily through the production of reactive oxygen species (ROS) and free radicals. These radicals damage parasitic proteins and membranes, leading to the rapid death of the malaria parasite. The endoperoxide bridge in the artesunate molecule is crucial for this activity.

Activity Against Parasite Stages: Artesunate is effective against multiple stages of the Plasmodium parasite's lifecycle, including the early ring stages and late schizonts. This broad-spectrum activity contributes to its efficacy in treating severe malaria.

2. Pharmacokinetics:

Absorption and Bioavailability: Artesunate is rapidly absorbed after administration, whether given intravenously, intramuscularly, or orally. It is quickly converted to its active metabolite, dihydroartemisinin (DHA), which is responsible for its antimalarial activity.

Distribution: After absorption, artesunate and DHA are widely distributed in body tissues, including the liver, kidneys, and brain. This extensive distribution is beneficial for targeting parasites in various organs.

Metabolism: Artesunate is rapidly hydrolyzed to DHA by plasma esterases. DHA is then further metabolized and eliminated primarily via the urine.

Elimination: The half-life of artesunate is short, typically less than one hour, while DHA has a half-life of about 1-2 hours. This rapid clearance necessitates frequent dosing or combination with longer-acting drugs.

3. Toxicology:

Acute Toxicity: Preclinical studies in animal models have shown that artesunate has a relatively high therapeutic index, meaning that it is effective at doses well below those that cause toxicity. However, at very high doses, artesunate can cause neurotoxicity, evidenced by degeneration of brainstem nuclei.

Chronic Toxicity: Long-term studies indicate that repeated doses of artesunate can cause hematological changes, such as decreased red and white blood cell counts. These effects are generally reversible upon discontinuation of the drug.

Reproductive Toxicity: Artesunate has shown teratogenic effects in animal studies, particularly during the first trimester of pregnancy. It can cause embryotoxicity, including resorptions and malformations, emphasizing the need for caution when prescribing to pregnant women.

4. Mutagenicity and Carcinogenicity:

Mutagenicity: Artesunate has not shown significant mutagenic potential in standard assays, such as the Ames test and chromosomal aberration tests.

Carcinogenicity: Long-term carcinogenicity studies have not demonstrated any significant increase in tumor formation associated with artesunate use.

Storage

Proper storage of artesunate is essential to maintain its efficacy and safety. Inappropriate storage conditions can lead to degradation of the active ingredient, reducing its therapeutic effectiveness.

1. General Storage Guidelines:

Temperature: Artesunate should be stored at controlled room temperature, typically between 15°C and 30°C (59°F and 86°F). It should be protected from excessive heat, which can cause degradation.

Humidity: Artesunate should be stored in a dry place, away from high humidity. Exposure to moisture can affect the stability of the lyophilized powder.

Light: Artesunate should be protected from light, as exposure can lead to photodegradation. It is usually stored in opaque or amber-colored vials to minimize light exposure.

2. Reconstituted Solution:

Shelf Life: Once reconstituted, artesunate solutions should be used immediately or stored at 2°C to 8°C (35.6°F to 46.4°F) and used within 24 hours. Prolonged storage of reconstituted solutions can lead to loss of potency.

Handling: Reconstituted artesunate should be handled aseptically to avoid contamination. Any unused solution should be discarded after 24 hours.

3. Stability:

Expiration Date: Artesunate products come with a labeled expiration date, beyond which the drug should not be used. This date is based on stability studies conducted under recommended storage conditions.

Packaging Integrity: The integrity of the packaging should be checked before use. Any signs of damage or contamination can compromise the sterility and efficacy of the drug.

Instructions

Proper instructions for the use of artesunate are critical for ensuring its safe and effective administration. Healthcare providers must be well-informed about these guidelines to provide the best care for patients.

1. Preparation:

Reconstitution: Artesunate is provided as a lyophilized powder that needs to be reconstituted with a sterile diluent, typically provided with the product. The exact amount of diluent and method of reconstitution should be followed as per the manufacturer's instructions.

Dilution: If further dilution is required for intravenous infusion, the reconstituted solution should be mixed with an appropriate volume of IV fluid (e.g., 5% dextrose or normal saline) to achieve the desired concentration.

2. Administration:

Intravenous Injection: The reconstituted solution can be administered as a slow IV injection over 1-2 minutes or as an infusion over 30 minutes to an hour. Proper aseptic technique should be used to avoid contamination.

Intramuscular Injection: For IM administration, the reconstituted solution should be injected deep into the muscle, preferably in the thigh or buttock. The injection should be given slowly to minimize pain and tissue damage.

3. Dosage:

Adult Dosage: The standard dosage for adults is 2.4 mg/kg body weight, administered initially at 0 hours, then at 12 and 24 hours, and subsequently once daily.

Pediatric Dosage: For children weighing less than 20 kg, the dosage is typically 3 mg/kg body weight, following the same administration schedule as adults.

4. Monitoring:

Clinical Monitoring: Patients should be closely monitored for clinical improvement, including the resolution of fever and reduction in parasite load. Blood smears or rapid diagnostic tests can be used to assess parasite clearance.

Adverse Effects: Monitoring for adverse effects, such as neurotoxicity, hematological changes, and allergic reactions, is essential. Regular blood counts and liver function tests may be required.

5. Patient Education:

Informing Patients: Patients and caregivers should be informed about the importance of completing the full course of treatment, potential side effects, and when to seek medical attention.

Follow-Up: Patients should be advised to return for follow-up visits to ensure complete parasite clearance and to monitor for any delayed adverse effects, such as hemolysis.

Presentation

Artesunate is available in various formulations and packaging, designed to facilitate its use in different clinical settings.

1. Formulations:

Lyophilized Powder: Artesunate is commonly supplied as a lyophilized powder for injection. This form is stable and has a longer shelf life, making it suitable for storage and transport to malaria-endemic regions.

Oral Tablets: Although less common, artesunate is also available in oral tablet form for use in combination therapies (ACTs) for uncomplicated malaria. These tablets are often co-formulated with other antimalarials, such as mefloquine or amodiaquine.

2. Packaging:

Vials: The lyophilized powder is typically packaged in single-dose vials, each containing a specific amount of artesunate (e.g., 60 mg).

These vials are accompanied by a sterile diluent for reconstitution.

Blister Packs: Oral tablets are usually packaged in blister packs, with each pack containing a full course of treatment. This packaging ensures the stability of the tablets and protects them from moisture and contamination.

3. Labeling:

Information: The packaging of artesunate products includes detailed labeling with important information such as the drug name, dosage form, concentration, storage conditions, expiration date, and instructions for reconstitution and administration.

Warnings: Labels also contain warnings about potential side effects, contraindications, and the need for careful monitoring, particularly in special populations such as pregnant women and patients with G6PD deficiency.

4. Accessibility:

Availability: Artesunate is widely available through various global health initiatives and programs aimed at improving access to effective malaria treatment in endemic regions. It is often provided to healthcare facilities in remote areas where malaria is prevalent.

Cost: Efforts to reduce the cost of artesunate and ensure its affordability are ongoing. Subsidies, donations, and bulk purchasing agreements help lower the price, making it accessible to low-income populations.

www.ingramcontent.com/pod-product-compliance
Lightning Source LLC
Chambersburg PA
CBHW071955210526
45479CB00003B/953